EMBODIMENT

The Manual You Should Have Been Given When You Were Born

Dr. Dain C. Heer

© by Dr. Dain C. Heer. All rights reserved.

Published by Lulu.com

ISBN: 978-0-557-41885-5

Standard Copyright License

Cover and Typesetting: Stephen Outram.

DR. DAIN HEER

Dr. Dain Heer has totally transformed his life through his work as an Access Consciousness Facilitator. Dain inspires and empowers others to access their infinite potential. He says "It's the weirdest thing I've ever found – and it is the most fun I have ever had!"

Although Dain is a qualified chiropractor, his work with Access Consciousness has allowed him to use bodywork techniques with results so dynamic that people start to enjoy greater freedom and ease with their bodies. To put into words what Dain is capable of facilitating with bodies is only a limitation; he is truly a gift.

Dr. Dain Heer regularly travels the world inspiring and assisting people to change their lives from the ordinary to extraordinary! He facilitates Access Consciousness seminars himself and also co-facilitates with Gary Douglas on a regular basis in the USA, Canada, Australia & New Zealand, Europe and more.

For more information about Dain please go to his website:

www.DrDainHeer.com

www.AccessConsciousness.com

CONTENTS

Embodiment   1

Introduction   11

You And Your Body   13
   What is oneness with the body?

Why Do You Have A Body   15
   How do you know what your body is saying to you?
   The Access Consciousness diet
   Have you denied your body what it has asked for?

Consciousness Includes Everything   22
   Allowance
   Interesting point of view

Humanoid Embodiment Vs Human Embodiment   26
   What's different about them?
   Humanoids look for ways to make things better
   This is all there is
   Humanoids tend to judge themselves
   Wait a minute!
   A four-foot fall from a running horse
   Yeah, yeah, that happened to somebody else

Humanoid Embodiment. What Are The Infinite Possibilities   33
   Your body has talents and abilities you haven't acknowledged
   Sometimes people suddenly step-out of human embodiment

Autopilot Vs Ten Second Increments   39

Your Body Is Your Animal   41

Caring   42
    What about helping your children to become more aware?
    You may have misapplied caring with your body

Follow The Energy – Don't Make It Significant   47
    Abuse
    Releasing the energy of abuse
    Affirmations

The Power In Caring   54
    Most of us only care for ourselves a tiny amount

Sexualness   57
    Embodying the sexualness of you
    Are you vibrantly alive and willing to receive the energy of the universe?

Sex, Sexualness, Sensualness, Copulation & Sexuality   61

The 1, 2, 3 Of Sex Vs The Communion Of Sexualness   64

Orgasm   68
    How many orgasms would your body like to have in a day?
    There's a false idea that orgasm is a completion

Everything In Your Life Should Be An Orgasmic Experience   72

Conversations With Bod. 10 Things Your Body Would Tell You If Only You'd Listen   74
    1. Do one thing a day to nurture, acknowledge and appreciate me
    2. Stop judging me
    3. I was created to have fun
    4. Ask me about me
    5. Ask me what it would take to get me to look the way you want me to

6. I'm the one eating
7. Ask me what movement I would like to do
8. Don't buy the latest fad
9. Ask, "Where does this come from?"
10. I'm a body and you're an infinite being

Have A Little Gratitude   85

Come out of judgment of yourself for not being perfect

A Note To Readers   90

INTRODUCTION

What if your body were an ongoing source of joy? What if you could enjoy your body the way cats, dogs or horses enjoy theirs? What if you got to move every muscle when you walked? What if every moment were an opportunity to lick yourself and purr? Could embodiment possibly be like that?

I'm a chiropractor by training; however, I'm interested in becoming an embodiment expert in practice, and helping you to become one, as well. Embodiment: The Manual You Should Have Been Given When You Were Born won't be like any other book on embodiment that you've ever read. It's not chiropractic. It's not medical. It's about functioning with your body from the perspective of beingness. It will explore how you, as an infinite being, can experience that greatness with your body.

This book may go against everything you've ever thought, everything you've been taught, and everything you've bought from everything and everyone else around you. It doesn't claim to give you the answers. Instead it will encourage you to ask questions. It will allow you to enjoy the body you currently have—and to enjoy the body you create.

The concepts in this book were discovered, in large part, through the work I've done with Gary Douglas, the founder of Access Consciousness, which is a modality that offers tools, information and processes to change any area of your life and encompass the greatness of your body. In the course of our ongoing collaboration, Gary and I have become aware that living the greatness of embodiment is a choice we all have—and it's my pleasure to share the tools for achieving that greatness in this book.

I'd like to express my gratitude for Gary, without whose extremely unique way of looking at the world, we wouldn't have this information.

Thanks for joining me.

Yours in joy,
Dr. Dain Heer

P.S. Please make sure to read the part subtitled, "If You're Expecting This to Be Endorsed by the Pope, Don't Read It."

YOU AND YOUR BODY

There are things your body is really good at, like eating, sleeping, having sex, and enjoying the feeling of the sun on its skin. These are your body's domains. This doesn't mean you're not there, too; you are, because you are oneness with your body. But it's important to realize that you are not your body. You're an infinite being who has a body.

Close your eyes and find the outside edges of you, the being. Not the outside edges of the body, but the outside edges of the being you are. Can you find the outside edges of you? Or is it more like wherever you go, there you are? You're everywhere. You exist within your body and outside of it at the same time. You as a being can't fit inside the yummy little vehicle called your body. You're too utterly enormous. No amount of force is going to make you fit inside your body.

What is oneness with the body?

When I speak of being in oneness, or communion with your body, I am talking about being in a place where you have no judgment about your body. When you're in oneness with it, there are no barriers between you and it. You're totally vulnerable with your body; you're completely present with it. You're willing to receive everything from it exactly as it is. But instead of being in communion with our bodies, most of us function from the antithesis of embodiment. We go against what embodiment could and should be. We ignore the infinite possibilities that we have available with these beautiful bodies of ours. the Greatness of embodiment Would you as a being come back to a body over and over again, lifetime after lifetime, if there weren't something great about embodiment? No. You wouldn't. If there weren't some greatness in embodiment, you would be saying, I'm done with this body. I'm going to find some way to un-create it so I can get the hell out of it. But this isn't what we do. We keep returning to bodies. There must be possibilities connected with having a body that we haven't tapped into.

I'd like to explore those possibilities with you in this book. I'd like to help you increase your awareness of your body so you know when it's communicating with you, and can hear what it's saying. Instead of having hit-and-miss communication like, "I think my body said it wanted peppers, but I don't know." you'll clearly get the message, "Hey, my body would like some … "

WHY DO YOU HAVE A BODY

You have a body to have fun. You have a body so you can feel the sun on your skin. So you can climb a tree. So you can experience the way the water feels when you walk into the ocean. So you can enjoy a soft caress when someone touches you gently. So you can taste sugar on the tongue, salt on the tongue, salt from someone's neck on your tongue.

Yesterday I did three sessions in the morning and I had a class to do in the evening. I was feeling tired and uncomfortable. I said, "Let me see. Body, what do you want to do?"

My body said, "Well, you've got two choices. You can either kill me now, or you can take me out for a jog and get me some sun and allow me to release a little of this energy you're holding onto."

I thought I was tired and needed a nap, but my body said, "We've got to get moving. You just think you need a nap. Come on, let's go."

I said, "Okay, cool."

How do you know what your body is saying to you?

Most of us don't ask our body anything. We assume we know what's right for it, or we do what other people tell us is good for it, but we don't check in with our bodies to see what they'd like. It's important to start asking your body what it wants. Ask it, "Body, what would you like to eat?" and you'll either get a picture of something your body would like, or it will lean towards something that it desires.

You can also muscle test your body to find out what it would like. Standing, put both of your feet together, toes and ankles, and hold the food or vitamin or whatever it is in front of your solar plexus and ask, "Body, would you like to ingest this?" If your body would like it, it will lean towards it. If it doesn't want it, it will lean away.

You can do this with all kinds of things: "Body, would you like to drink this?" "Body, lean forward when you get to the amount you want." If you just stand there, heels and toes together, your body will respond. You can also do this with clothing: hold a piece of clothing out in front of your belly, and ask, "Body, would you like to wear this?"

Your body will let you know what it likes. You'll find that there are certain things your body likes to wear. There are certain materials it likes. If you'll ask, your body will tell you.

When I first started facilitating Access classes, Gary Douglas, Access' founder, said to me, "You have a great body. You need to show it off." At the time I was wearing the equivalent of male muumuus; extra large shirts with an undershirt underneath and the baggiest pants you've ever seen. I hadn't bought new clothes in years.

When Gary said, "You need to show off your body,"

I said, "This body?"

He said, "Yes."

So I bought clothes I thought were sexy and showed off my body. I got a lot of close-fitting Kenneth Cole polyester shirts. They were an improvement over what I had been wearing, however, when I put them on my body, it wasn't happy. I wasn't quite aware of it, though. Then one day when I was shopping, I went into Banana Republic and I saw a linen shirt. My body fell over itself to get to it. It said, "Oh wow, I love this shirt. This is the kind of clothing you want to wear, okay?"

It was the linen. My body loved the linen. I put the shirt on and I looked in the mirror and I said, "Whoa!" My whole body shifted and changed. It was saying, "Yes, I'm here and I'm happy, and thank God you are buying this and getting rid of your polyester." There are things your body takes joy in. Wouldn't it be great to become aware of what those things are?

In the morning, you can open your closet and ask your body, "Body, what would you like to wear today?" Or you can ask the clothes which ones would like to be worn. When you happen to find a match between what your body would like to wear and the clothing that would like to be worn, those are the days when you'll be looking good and strutting your stuff. How does this work? Your body desired it and the clothing said, "Hey, I can provide that for you." Everything has consciousness, including your body and your clothes.

Just stand in front of your closet and ask, "Body, what would you like to wear today?" Your body will either lean or turn towards something or you'll just see the item and know. You might decisively grab something and say, Oh, I'll wear that! It's simple. Remember, you're starting something new. You may not be perfect at first, and you may not get an answer the same way twice. But start opening up to the awareness of your body, and what it would like, in every area of your life.

Asking what your body would like can be particularly effective if you would like to lose weight. I know a lady in Santa Barbara who came over from Australia to do more Access, and she got married. She's been asking her body what it wants and over the past six months she has lost over 150 pounds. Guess what she's been eating? She's been eating anything her body wants, which sometimes includes junk food, and she's been having a lot of sex. She's been enjoying her life. Isn't that cool?

The Access Consciousness diet

If you ask your body what it wants, it may be junk food. Yesterday I had several bowls of Corn Pops. I had Doritos. I asked, "Body, are you sure you want this?"

It said, "Oh yeah."

I had some Celtic sea salt straight out of the container. I was thinking to myself, My goodness, what a strange day for my body. Last night at dinner time, I asked, "Body, what would you like?"

It wanted a fish sandwich. So I snorted that right down and it was good, and I felt great.

When I woke up this morning, I felt like I needed to sleep a bit longer, so I slept until the last possible moment. My body wanted food, but I was running late. My body wanted me to eat before I gave a session, but I didn't have time. As it worked out, I didn't eat for five hours, and my body was not happy with me. It was saying, "You need to eat. I told you to eat. I asked you to eat. Now you're not feeling so good, are you? Neither am I."

After I finally got some food and gave it what it wanted, it felt great again.

You can also ask your body about vitamins and supplements. I used to consume around $300 a month worth of vitamins, trying to get my body to feel good. I'll take these herbs. I'll take this liquid supplement. I'll take this salt. I'll do this, I'll do that. I would read something that described my symptoms and I'd think, Okay, this describes my symptoms. It will probably take care of them.

In truth, the only thing that's going to take care of you is consciousness and awareness of your body. Stop trying to get results with every fad you hear about. Be in communion with your body, and your body will tell you when something comes along that it desires.

We talked about this at a class in New York and one of the participants asked her body, "Hey Body, what would it take for us to lose this excess body fat?" And then she just went about her life.

A few days later she overheard someone she didn't know talking about a diet. She walked over and said, "I'm sorry, I don't mean to interrupt, but I hear you talking about this diet. Can you tell me about it?"

The woman told her about it and it was exactly what her body wanted. She did that diet and ended up losing 50 pounds in a matter of weeks. Why? Because it was what her body asked for.

Have you denied your body what it has asked for?

Have you denied your body what it has asked for and done it with such vehemence that now you have no idea what it wants? You can change this. Here is what you need to do. First of all, say: I revoke, recant, rescind, reclaim, renounce, destroy and un-create all that I've done to deny what my body has asked for.

Then, ask your body what it would like. Listen to what it says and do what it tells you.

People have asked me, "Do you mean I should use this with everything? Do you mean I should ask my body rather than listening to myself?"

And I say, "Yes, for everything that involves your body." This includes anything you're going to put in your body or anything you're going to do with it. "Body, who would you like to have sex with? Body, who would you like to play with? Body, who would you like to have massage you?"

You wouldn't pull over to the side of the road and pour dirt into your gas tank and expect your car to run. But you eat all kinds of shit your body has no desire to eat. You eat ten times the amount it wants. You don't drink enough water. You take all of those supplements that your body has no desire or need for, and you are making it sick, all because you read some article, or some idiot, who had no idea what your body wanted, told you it was going to help. Don't listen to anybody about your body, other than your body.

Ask your body about things that concern it. "Hey body, what would you like?" For example, do you exercise—or does your body exercise? Your body does. You might have some exercise in mind for your body, and it might be thinking, "I don't think so. Do I want to do that? No." So ask it, "Body, what movement would you like?" And when it answers you, do the movement it requests. You can't just think about it in your head. You have to actually move your body. Your body's point of view is, "I want to have my limbs and my parts moving, okay?"

Someone asked me, "What if your body doesn't want to go to the office?"

In a situation like this, you can ask, "Okay body, what can we do or change that would allow you to be more comfortable and more at ease in the office?"

There are going to be things that you have to do regardless of what your body desires. When that's the case, ask, "Hey Body, how can we make this easier on you? How can we have this be more fun? What would it take for that?"

Your body might say, "Lots of alcohol." I doubt it would ask for this, but if it does, you should probably do it. Your body's saying, "I'll be a lot happier without perceiving all the crap these people are trying to throw at you. Just get me schnockered."

CONSCIOUSNESS INCLUDES EVERYTHING

At the completion of the Access Level Two and Three classes, Gary Douglas used to channel an entity named Raz. People asked Raz questions, and Gary channelled his replies.

There was a lady in one of the classes who was talking about all the sad things that were going on in her life and she asked to speak with Raz.

She said, "Raz, I'm so sad. I can't handle all the pain and suffering. It's horrendous."

Raz asked, "Would there be suffering in oneness?"

She said, "No."

He said, "Really? There wouldn't be suffering in oneness? Would there be sadness in oneness?"

She said, "No."

He said, "Really? There wouldn't be any sadness in oneness? Doesn't oneness include everything and judge nothing?"

Oneness is synonymous with consciousness; it includes everything. It includes every possibility you could imagine without any judgment. It includes every greatness possible. It also includes all the pain, suffering, trauma and drama people choose.

You have a white flower and a red flower. Which is better? Hello? You don't do that to flowers. You have somebody crying and somebody laughing. Which is better? Who's to say?

Whatever you choose is okay, but be aware that people who say they're choosing consciousness are usually choosing their own version of a polarized reality. A polarized reality contains concepts like good and evil, happy and sad, beautiful and ugly. Most of us think we're choosing consciousness, when in reality we're still caught up in our preferences, opinions and judgments. We say we're choosing consciousness, but we're beating the shit out of other people. We say outrageous things like, Because I'm choosing consciousness, I can see where you're being an asshole to everyone around you.

Guess what? If you have that point of view, you are functioning from a more polarized reality than the person you're judging. Doing Access does not mean you're choosing consciousness. Please understand that. Choosing consciousness is the only proof that you're choosing consciousness. There's no room for being in judgment of anyone or anything.

If you have a judgment of someone else, if you have a judgment of your body, if you have a judgment of your wife, if you have a judgment of your husband, if you have a judgment of your kids, if you have a judgment of your car, it's time to get over it. You don't have the luxury of limiting yourself with judgment. You can't do it. You have too much power.

How do you get over it? You go into allowance.

Allowance

Notice that you're judging: Oh, I'm judging that? Then go into allowance. When you move into allowance, or a place of no judgment, you recognize that you are everything and you judge nothing, including yourself. There is simply no judgment in your universe. There is total allowance of all things.

When you are in allowance, you are a rock in the stream. Thoughts, ideas, beliefs, attitudes and emotions come at you, and they go around you and you are still the rock in the stream. Everything is an interesting point of view.

Acceptance is different from allowance. If you are in acceptance, when thoughts, ideas, beliefs and attitudes come at you and you are in the stream, you get washed away. In acceptance, you either align and agree, which is the positive polarity, or you resist and react, which is the negative polarity. Either way, you get washed away.

Interesting point of view

If you are in allowance of what I'm saying, you can say, Well, that's an interesting point of view. I wonder if there's any truth in that. You go into a question instead of a reaction.

How is this in everyday life? You and your friend are walking down the street and she says to you, "I look awful today!" What do you do?

"Oh, you poor thing! You do look tired. You're working too much!" is alignment and agreement.

"No, you don't! You look great!" is resistance and reaction.

Interesting point of view is, "Really? What makes you say that?"

You can use interesting point of view as an approach to every aspect of your life. Does someone or something irritate you? He, she or it is not the problem. You are. As long as you have any irritation, you've got a problem. It's not about the way others respond to you. It's about you being in allowance of them as completely bat-shit as they are.

You don't have to align and agree with them, nor do you have to resist and react to them. Neither of those is real. You simply allow, honor and respect their point of view without buying it. Being in allowance of somebody doesn't mean you have to be a doormat. You just have to be with what is.

The hardest thing is to be in allowance of yourself. We tend to judge and judge and judge ourselves. We get locked into trying to be a good parent or a good partner or a good whatever and we're always judging ourselves. But we can be in allowance of our own point of view. We can say, I had that point of view. Interesting. I did that. Interesting.

If you truly desire to create and enjoy the possibilities of embodiment, there's no room for limiting yourself with judgment anymore. There's no room for projecting judgment onto your body. There's no room for projecting it on other people. Go into allowance: Oh, wasn't that interesting she'd choose that? I don't know why she'd choose it but okay, cool. Gee, I had that judgment about myself or my body? Isn't that interesting?

HUMANOID EMBODIMENT VS HUMAN EMBODIMENT

We have two majorly different perspectives and ways of creating here on Planet Earth: we have the human perspective and the humanoid perspective. The human perspective is that force is the source of creation. Humans think you have to work hard and sweat in order to create things. This is not so for humanoids. Humanoids recognize their oneness with the universe, and they don't pit themselves against it.

What's different about them?

Our investigation into humans and humanoids began on a trip Gary and I took to Nashville. Gary is always trying to figure out how to help get people out of their shit and what's limiting them, and the way he does this is to walk into their space and look at the maze. He finds the route out of the maze, and then he can figure out how to help people resolve it.

We were in our seats on the plane and two women walked down the aisle and sat down in front of us. Gary said, "I wonder what it would take to free somebody like that," and he went into their heads. I was saying, "Don't go in! Don't go in!" but it was too late. He was in there going, "Uhhh," and I had to work on him for 45 minutes to get him out of their universe. He was trying to find a way out, only there was none. Their maze was closed.

The ladies took off their jackets and put them over the seats in front of them and when the stewardess came by and said, "Here's your lunch," they put it in their laps.

Embodiment. The Manual You Should Have Been Given When You Were Born

When the stewardess asked, "Would you like a drink?" One of the ladies said, "Well, I have no place to put my drink."

The stewardess said, "Put your tray table down."

The lady said, "I don't have a tray table."

The stewardess said, "See this man here sitting next to you? That thing down there, that's your tray table."

The lady said, "I don't have one."

The stewardess said, "If you will take your jacket off the back of the seat ..."

The lady said, "I'm not putting my jacket on the floor."

Gary was saying, "Oh shit, how did I get in here? How do I get out?" It wasn't until he asked, "Okay, what's different about these people? How are they different from Dain and me and the people we work with in Access? What's different about them?" that he got it: "They're so human! Oh my God. We're different. We're not human. What are we? We're humanoid! I can't believe this. I've been thinking I'm human all this time and I'm not. I'm humanoid."

He got free by understanding that he wasn't one of them. It took the recognition that he wasn't like them.

We have known people like those ladies all our lives, and we have always tried to understand where they were coming from. We hadn't realized there were two species of beings on planet Earth. This was very helpful information.

Humanoids look for ways to make things better

Humans live in judgment of everybody else and think that life is just the way it is, and nothing is ever right, so don't even bother to think about another possibility. Humanoids, on the other hand, look for ways to make things better. If you invent things, if you search out things, if you are always looking for a better, bigger way of creating something, you're a humanoid. Humanoids are the people who create change. They create the inventions, the music and the poetry. They create all the things that come out of a lack of satisfaction with the status quo.

This is all there is

Gary visited his step-dad, who was very definitely human, after he had a heart attack. He said, "Dad, what was it like for you having that heart attack?" Nobody had asked him that question.

Gary's step-dad said, "Well, I remember having the heart attack and standing outside my body looking at it...." He trailed off and then started over again.

"Well, I had the heart attack and then I saw them putting the electrodes on my chest...." Again, he stopped mid-sentence, waited a moment, and then started over again.

"Well," he finally said, "I had the heart attack and then they put the electrodes on my chest and they zapped me."

He could not have a reality in which he was out of his body watching these things occur. It was a great example of what happens to people when they can't have what doesn't fit their judgments of reality. His reality was that you are a body and that's all there is. A human can never have anything that doesn't match the viewpoint, "This is all there is."

Humans are the people who do not believe in reincarnation. They do not believe in other possibilities. They do not believe in miracles or magic. The doctors and the lawyers and the Indian chiefs create everything. Humans create nothing.

Forty-seven percent of the population is humanoid and they are the creators of everything that changes in this reality. Fifty-two percent is human. (And the final one percent? Some day we'll tell you about them!) Humans hold onto things the way they are and never want anything to change. Have you ever been to somebody's house where they haven't changed the furniture in thirty years? Human.

Humanoids tend to judge themselves

One of the big differences between humans and humanoids is that humanoids tend to judge themselves, and humans judge others. You may, as a humanoid, occasionally try to judge others, but usually you only do that when trying to make yourself more like humans. Judging others is hard work for you. Most humanoids find it impossible. When they hear a judgment of someone, they say, "Huh? That would be important based on what? So-and-so did that? Well, maybe under certain circumstances so would I." A human, on the other hand, will say with great certainty, "No, I would never do that."

Instead of sitting in judgment of others, humanoids tend to sit in judgment of themselves. They find fault with themselves. They try to figure out how to make themselves better. A human doesn't do this. A human will tell you what's wrong with you, and how if you just did things differently or if you would just get in line with everybody else, everything would be okay. "If you'd just stop doing all those weird things you do," they say, "you'd be just fine. And why would you want anything better than what you've got, anyway, because this is all there is?" That's pretty much their defining point of view.

This is not so for humanoids. Humanoids recognize their oneness with their bodies and the world around them. They're willing to be in communion with their bodies, and as a result, the possibilities of embodiment show up for them.

Wait a minute!

Gary worked with a man in Australia who had Guillain-Barré Syndrome. It's a condition where a person's muscles literally atrophy. The man's legs looked like pancakes with two sticks through them. Gary did a hands-on process on the man's feet and he showed the man's wife and friend how to do it on his entire body. He spent three hours with them, and when he left the man's legs looked normal again. Not only that, but the man had been unable to move.

As Gary was leaving, the man was using the phone for the first time in weeks, and when he sneezed, he covered his mouth with his hand. A major change. We hear about things like this and we say, Wait a minute! We realize that the limitations we have bought about embodiment have to be a lie. The rate at which the body can heal is far greater than we had thought. Its possibilities are far greater than we have been led to believe. We have all heard stories like these. And most often people say, Oh yeah, right. They're full of crap. But what if we didn't discount the stories? Instead, what if we looked into—and changed—the belief systems that create our limited and unhappy points of view about embodiment?

A four-foot fall from a running horse

When we were in Costa Rica doing an Access workshop, our friend Cristina fell off a horse that was cantering. She landed face first in the mud and her body was in shock. As far as Gary and I could tell, her jaw was fractured or broken, and her wrist or her elbow was displaced. I held her for a minute or two, and began taking away everything that was creating those injuries in her body. Gary came a few minutes later and he held her and took out the rest, and another friend joined us. All of us worked on her that day in class.

By the end of the day Cristina had some marks on her face, but she didn't have any pain, she could chew soft foods, and the alignment on her jaw was about 99 percent. Two days later, she didn't have any black and blue marks at all, her jaw was perfectly aligned, and she was ready to chew anything again. She was dancing at the party we had that evening.

When somebody falls from a running horse, that's a four-foot fall to the ground. We could perceive what had happened structurally to her body and the amount of shock it was in. There was nobody home. But by the time Gary and I were done holding her, she had come home again. That she had no pain was a miracle. That's an example of the enormous possibilities that come with being in communion with our bodies.

Cristina says that experience changed a lot of things for her. She had been skeptical about energy and healing work, so the universe had to literally hit her in the face pretty damn hard to change her mind and get her moving.

Yeah, yeah, that happened to somebody else

A lady whose husband had third stage bone cancer called Gary and said, "What can I do?" Gary and I had recently discovered that when I worked on Gary's joints, it seemed to increase the ability of his immune system to function. So he said, "Well, we just found a new way of working with the body," and he described the process we were doing, which is about changing the blueprint of the body. He told her to do it on her husband's joints.

She did it on him every day—and eight weeks later when they checked him at the hospital, they said he was in total remission from third stage bone cancer. Third stage bone cancer is the stage right before they buy your casket. They had expected him to be in fourth stage and they were planning a treatment regimen, which he never required.

These things are possible, and yet often we will not allow them into our awareness. We adopt a human perspective. We hear about these miracles and possibilities, and we say, Yeah, yeah, that happened to somebody else.

The problem is that if you don't claim the totality of your humanoid capacity, you try to create from a human point of view. You believe in—and create—a limited possibility for yourself. How much of what's possible with your body have you cut out of your awareness? How many of the possibilities of humanoid embodiment have you totally dismissed with, Yeah, yeah, that happened to someone else?

The idea of bringing up the differences between humans and humanoids is not about sitting in judgment of humans. It's about becoming aware that we have an infinite capacity to experience the greatness of embodiment rather than buying into the limited human perspective that is all around us.

HUMANOID EMBODIMENT. WHAT ARE THE INFINITE POSSIBILITIES

I have discovered something very interesting about my body. It can almost instantaneously change its shape and size. At first, even when I saw it happening, I didn't believe it. It happened to me probably 100 times before I believed that it was actually occurring, and could say, Okay, it's happening.

Gary and I used to go to the gym to do our workouts together. One day when we were working out, I realized he was looking down at me and I was looking up at him, which is okay—except that Gary and I are about the same height. We're just about eye-to-eye. Yet here he was, looking down at me. Every time we went to work out, I noticed that I was four inches shorter than he was.

I thought, This is ridiculous. There is no way he is four inches taller than I am. We're the same height! I tried various ways to explain it. I'd say, Well, no, he's really only two inches taller than I am. But when we'd stand shoulder to shoulder at the gym, I could clearly see that he was at least four inches taller.

One day he asked me, "Did you used to work out with guys that were taller than you?"

I said, "Yeah, all the time." And instantaneously we were eye-to-eye again. The same height. I didn't move a muscle. I didn't shift my stance. I didn't think, Oh now I'm going to rise from the ashes. I will now get taller. I didn't think anything. I just grew four inches and returned to my regular height.

As I thought about it, I realized that when we worked out together, my body returned to the place it knew I worked out from: That was a place where my workout partners were guys that were taller than I was. So my body made an adjustment: It got four inches shorter every time I'd go to the gym. It did what it needed to do to make Gary taller than I was, just like the guys I used to work out with.

Growing four inches like that? That's impossible, right? I'm here to tell you it's not impossible. Yeah, yeah, that happened to somebody else.

This isn't the only time my body has spontaneously changed its shape and size. The brother of a friend of mine came to visit me from Australia, and I noticed that I was shorter than he was. I had been working out quite a bit at the time and my body was quite built up, but when I got around him, my body became smaller. My shirts suddenly got bigger. I observed this happening and asked myself, What the heck is going on? It happened whenever I was in this guy's presence.

He was a 19-year old Australian kid, visiting the United States for the first time. He was insecure, unhappy, and felt really bad about himself. When I was around him, my body became smaller. My shirts got baggy. My body would shrink to make him feel better about himself. Nice body. Way to go. Very kind.

I would leave his presence and ask myself, "Who did that belong to?" and I could feel my shirt on my skin again. Holy shit. Are you supposed to be able to change the size of your body just like that? I thought it was impossible. Yeah, yeah, that happened to somebody else.

When Gary first saw these changes happening and recognized them for what they were, he started telling people about it. I'd say, "Shhh ... Don't tell them that. That's not true. They're not going to believe it." You're not supposed to be able to change your body just like that. I could see it was happening to my body, but I wouldn't acknowledge it was true.

With humanoid embodiment there are a lot of things that can be different from what we have allowed ourselves to believe. If my body can grow four inches and shrink four inches—if it can go four inches this way and three inches this way, just like that—what are the possibilities for humanoid embodiment that we haven't allowed ourselves to consider?

Your body has talents and abilities you haven't acknowledged

I'm not sharing this with you so you'll think I'm cool. I want you to look at what you body will do. Your body probably has talents and abilities you haven't acknowledged. Let's take out the probably. Your body has talents and abilities you haven't acknowledged.

I was as surprised and perplexed by what my body did as anybody else would be. I couldn't believe it at first, and still might not, if Gary hadn't been there, observing it with me. It's not the bone structure. It's not the muscle structure. It's not the veins. It's not the arteries. It's not the heart. It's not all the things we think create the structure of our bodies. It's consciousness.

Gary and I were in New Zealand a while ago to teach some classes, and while we were there, we were doing a clearing process on some areas of my life where I had been disempowering myself. In the midst of that, a dramatic shift took place. We said, "Okay, cool." And that was the end of that.

The next morning, I went to put on my pants and they were way too big. I had lost almost two inches in my waist. I took the pants over to Gary and said, "Do you want a pair of pants—because these don't fit me any more. They're done."

When I walked into the class we were teaching, somebody who hadn't seen me for a while said, "Oh my God, what happened to you? How long have you been working out to get that result?"

I said, "Well, it happened in a split second with an Access process."

He said, "I don't know what you're doing but I want to do it, too."

Sometimes people suddenly step-out of human embodiment

Sometimes people suddenly step-out of human embodiment and move into humanoid embodiment. A lady told me she had an interesting dream one night and when she woke up every cell in her body was on. She felt like she had lifted off from the bed and come back down onto it, and her body buzzed with energy for at least half an hour.

Since then she's had other, similar episodes, not quite as intense as the first one, where great amounts of energy move through every cell of her body, and the body itself becomes much more present. When she described this to me, she said she knew it was not a human experience of embodiment.

I agreed that it was definitely not a human experience of embodiment and asked her to claim, own and acknowledge it as an awareness of humanoid embodiment. Sometimes we have moments where we step out of being human. We perceive our bodies vibrating or perceive the space between the molecules of the body. It's important to claim and own those as moments where we have stepped out of being human. They are the beginnings of humanoid embodiment.

Humanoid embodiment can be like having an orgasm past the orgasm. If you're going to create a body as a humanoid, is it going to be pain and suffering or is it going to be fun and joy? Fun and joy, right? If you're not having fun with your body, you're doing some version of the human limitation of embodiment—not humanoid embodiment.

When you notice yourself doing human limitations, you can say, Oops, I must have been wrong, then destroy and uncreate them and choose again. If what you're doing with your body isn't fun, if it's not joyful, if it's on autopilot, you're not being aware and present with your body.

The more of humanoid embodiment that I've claimed and owned, the easier and more fun my life has become. We often don't speak about our experiences of humanoid embodiment; usually these are the sorts of things that people keep to themselves. If they do have these experiences, they usually don't mention them until we ask about it in a class, and people will say, "Yeah, I have those experiences."

Has anything like this happened to you? How many times have you cut off something you could do because other people said it wasn't possible? What could we really have and how could we really be if we allowed ourselves to be and have all that was possible?

All of the talents, abilities and awareness that you decided you couldn't ever have again, will you now claim, own and acknowledge them, and destroy and uncreate everything that doesn't allow them to exist?

This journey you're embarking on with your body is one that people have avoided for centuries. Are you willing to be among the first to claim and own the possibilities of humanoid embodiment? I'm sorry. You may end up being different from your friends. Is that okay with you?

AUTOPILOT VS TEN SECOND INCREMENTS

Most of us live our lives on autopilot. Have you noticed that? We move through our lives on autopilot and come out of it only when there's a problem, and we have to look at it to shift and change it. We shake ourselves out of autopilot and ask, Okay, what is this? or Okay, how do I get rid of this?

On the other side of autopilot is living in ten-second increments. Each ten seconds of life is new. You get to choose what it's going to be. If you do everything in your life in ten-second increments, you will find you cannot make a wrong decision. You get angry for ten seconds and get over it. You love someone for ten seconds. You can love anyone for that amount of time, no matter who they are. You can hate someone for ten seconds. You can divorce your spouse for ten seconds. And you can love him or her in the next ten. If you live in ten-second increments, you create being in the present moment.

Rather than living in the moment, most people go on autopilot—or they try to create a plan and a system for the future, based on making the "right" choice or decision that will handle everything forever. But there's only one place we can live and that's right here, right now. Anything else kills us. We don't get to have a life. We miss out on our own life.

If you practice the art of choosing your life in ten-second increments you will begin to create choice and awareness.

If you had ten seconds to choose the rest of your life, what would you choose? Wealth? Okay, that ten seconds is over.

You've got ten seconds to live the rest of your life—what do you choose? Laughter? Joy? Consciousness?

Do you see how autopilot and ten-second increments of choice are mutually exclusive? If you're doing autopilot, you're not doing choice. If you're doing choice, you're not doing autopilot.

How many autopilot systems do you have for creating your body? What happens to you when you wake up in the morning? Do you immediately go into autopilot and do your morning routine? Instead, what about choosing humanoid embodiment for ten seconds? And then another ten. And another?

On a potential humanoid embodiment day, you wake up, you perceive the bed you're lying in and the softness of the sheets. You smell your own soft scent on the pillow and the scent of whoever is sleeping next to you. You perceive the warmth of the sun shining in the windows. You not only feel it, but you can perceive the vibration of it with your body. Then you make a choice for the next ten seconds. What will it be?

Sounds like a pretty cool way to start the day, don't you think?

This level of perception and awareness is not something that you're necessarily going to step right into, but you can step into a lot of it. It takes practice. You have to be willing to have humanoid embodiment and you have to be willing to have awareness. You have to be willing to develop total awareness of this beautiful thing called your body. Are you willing?

YOUR BODY IS YOUR ANIMAL

Have you ever had an animal that loves you unconditionally, that cares for you so much that it doesn't matter what you do? It doesn't matter if you're an absolute ass-hole. It doesn't matter if you yell at it. It is always there for you. For me, it's my horse. He's there for me all the time.

Can you imagine what it would be like if you allowed your communion with your body to be like that? You've got a very intelligent animal. You're connected with it intimately in every way. It's your body. Would you claim and own the communion and connection with your body that is possible and that is the truth of you? When you do feel that communion, it's always joy and peace. You have a very joyful and peaceful body, if you will allow it to be.

CARING

True caring is acknowledging the infinite choice that each individual has. True caring is being willing to allow another person to make choices even if you think those choices might hurt them. It's being willing to allow someone that you care about to choose to leave their body if that's their choice. That's true caring.

Most people have misidentified and misapplied what caring means. They think caring means something like: I'll try to stop you from doing anything that I think might hurt you, and if I can't stop you then I'll judge you, because I care about you.

Have you ever had your parents do that? My mom cares about me so much, and when I told her I was learning to jump with my horse over fences, she said, "Oh my God, be careful! You could fall and get hurt." I was going out for my first jumping lesson with my horse, nervous already, thank you very much, and she said, "Oh be careful because you could fall and get hurt."

Guess what? I fell. I've fallen off horses four other times, but this was the only time I've fallen that I haven't landed on my feet. It was the only time I landed smack flat on the ground. My helmet came over onto my face and rubbed off all the skin on my nose, and guess what? I was pissed at my mother. Isn't that interesting? I got mad at my mother instead of asking myself, Why did I buy that shit? What was I doing?

I bought her point of view that I could get hurt by jumping with my horse over fences. Excuse me. I can get hurt by jumping with my horse? If I'm in total awareness, am I going to get hurt doing anything? No. I'd have the awareness not to do something that was going to hurt me. I'd have the awareness not to go there.

Mothers have told me when their kids are going to do something they think is risky, the first thing that hits them is the fear their kid will get hurt. I ask them, "Is that fear your point of view, yes or no?" and they always reply, "No."

It's a point of view they've learned through years of being a mother, through a long line of mothers who bred guilt and fear into their children in an effort to protect them from getting hurt.

I ask mothers, "Do guilt and fear prevent your kids from getting hurt or do they actually create a greater possibility of them hurting themselves?" They pretty much always agree that guilt and fear of getting hurt aren't helpful. So, I ask them, "What would be a different choice?"

What about helping your children to become more aware?

You can do this by asking them questions: Hey honey, how does that feel to you? Does it feel exciting? Is there anything about it that's not exciting? Is there any heaviness about it? Is there anything you're worried about? No? Cool, have a great time. That's the difference you can create when you encourage awareness and ask questions.

When I told my mom I was going to jump with my horse over fences, she didn't encourage me to be aware. She didn't ask, "Hey, are you excited?"

I would have said, "Yeah!"

She didn't ask, "Are you worried about it at all?"

I would have said, "I'm having a great time. I'm looking forward to this. My horse kicked off its back shoes because he wants to jump so badly. I think we'll have fun."

She didn't ask a question. She didn't encourage awareness. Instead, she slammed me with her point of view. This was misidentified as caring. But caring is not about imposing your point of view or controlling the shit out of everyone you love to make sure they do what you've decided is best for them.

If you look at a situation from the truth of caring, which is more empowering—asking questions—or imposing a point view on someone? What do you want to do with your kids? Do you want to impose your point of view on them and have them buy it? Or would you rather ask them questions that encourage them to be aware of what they're doing?

I have a friend whose daughter went to live in Mexico and the girl's mother kept saying to her, "Be careful, darling. Be careful. Be careful." The daughter called her dad and said, "Dad, what should I do? Mom is driving me nuts with this 'be careful' stuff."

He said to her, "Honey, it's more important to be aware than it is to be careful. Being careful comes from the idea that everything is going to be bad. Being aware simply means you are aware of the energy. Feel the energy of a situation and you'll stay out of trouble. Don't try to protect yourself by being careful. Take care of yourself by being aware."

Several months later, after his daughter had returned to the U.S., she called him one night and said, "Dad, call me and tell me I have to come home right now. Things are not feeling right at this party. There are three drunk guys here and six more on the way, and there are only three girls. Call me and tell me I have to come home."

That's being aware. That's the kind of result you can create by teaching your kids to ask questions and to be aware—rather than careful.

You may have misapplied caring with your body

You may have done this with your body. You may have decided something like this: I care about my body, so I will have it do everything I've decided is best for it. I'm going to have some more ozone now without ever asking you what you would like, body. Here, body, swallow some more fish oil.

There are times, for example, when you might wake up in the morning and think you're tired, and if that's your point of view, you'll impose it on your body. But instead of doing that, what if you asked your body a question? "Hey body, are you tired?" It might say, "No, I feel fine. I got eight hours of sleep. You, the being, were out last night playing around or working—or whatever it is that you do—so that's why you think we should be tired. But I'm not tired. I feel great."

The important thing is asking your body. Caring doesn't come from a decision or a point of view; it comes from asking your body what it desires and being willing to honor its request. If your body says, "I don't want to take these vitamin pills any more," even if you've been taking them for 25 years, you'll be willing to listen to it and honor its request.

I've been feeling tired lately because we've been doing so much work without any real time off, and this morning when I got up, I had the thought, I want to go jogging.

I asked my body, "Do you want to go jogging?"

It said, "Yeah! Let's go."

So I went out for just a little while, and it was really energizing to me even though I woke up with the idea that I was tired. It was a lot more caring to ask my body what it needed and to listen to its request, rather than assume I knew what was best for it.

FOLLOW THE ENERGY – DON'T MAKE IT SIGNIFICANT

One of the great things I've learned as an Access practitioner is to follow the energy of the person I'm working with and not to make anything significant. It doesn't matter what kind of energy it is, physical energy, emotional energy, or mental energy. I've learned to regard it as simply an interesting point of view. The energy comes up, I follow it, and it releases. I'll notice there's a lot of energy on something and I'll say, Oh, wow. Lot of energy on that. I'll just acknowledge it's there.

When I first started out as an Access practitioner, I used to make other people's emotions, especially sadness, very significant. Oh dear Lord, the overwhelming sadness of it all. We tend to be very good at perceiving or picking up on the emotions, feelings, thoughts or points of view of the people we grew up around. We tend to recognize them all the time in everyone and everything around us. As a kid, I grew up around two things: deep sadness and huge amounts of suppressed anger, and I'm great at perceiving those, wherever I happen to be.

Once when I was in Australia, I was doing bodywork on someone who had a great deal of sadness locked up in her body, and I was helping her release it. As I worked with her, I could perceive her sadness intensely and it was so overwhelming to me that I was crying.

Working with her in this way required a great deal of energy, and I was exhausted afterwards. Later, I told Gary about it. He has a wonderful way of throwing a dagger into your reality when you're not expecting it. He calls it his Wedge Technique. He throws in a wedge and your door never shuts the same again. He asked, "Were you making any part of that sadness significant?"

I said, "Oh yes! I was so significant about the sadness."

He said, "Well, how did you feel after you did that session?"

I said, "I was drained. There was so much sadness. It was difficult to deal with."

Then he asked, "Did making the sadness significant assist you to help that person? Did it expand—or did it contract—what you were able to do with her?"

As soon as he asked the question, I realized that I had made the sadness significant and the result was that I was much less effective in helping her than I could have been. I said, "Okay. I'm not making emotion significant anymore."

Not long after that, when I was working on another person, a similar emotion came up and I asked myself two questions: What would happen if I didn't make this emotion significant? and What are the infinite possibilities for shifting this emotion? I had no clue how it was going to happen.

As I worked with this person, I had my hand on him, in a very similar place to the first person, and the same emotion came up. There was a great deal of energy, but this time I wasn't attaching the emotion of sadness to it, and I wasn't making it significant. The most interesting thing happened. I started laughing. I started laughing and the energy moved on through this person's body and released. He got at least 100 times more benefit from our session than the first person got.

It takes a huge amount of energy to make something significant, and in doing so you have to constrict it, which inhibits its release. To let it go, you just have to take the significance away and let it be light. You don't have to make anything significant, and if you don't make people's energy or their emotion significant, they won't drain you.

My mother started doing Access after I got over the point of view that I wanted her to do it. When she started, she was very significant about her sadness. She's a wonderful woman. I love her dearly. But she sounded like she was dying all the time and she was always so friggin' sad and wasn't even aware of it. She thought she was happy, but I could perceive the sadness.

When I stopped making her sadness significant, she stopped being so sad. I had been thinking, If I just go into this once more and find out why she's sad, I can get her out of having to be sad. But what I was really doing was making the sadness significant, real and solid, and that kept her in it more. Things changed for the better as soon as I let go of the significance.

What emotion have you made real, Intense and significant?

What emotion did you grow up with that you have made real, intense and significant? Rejection? Anxiety? Depression? Guilt? Or was it something else? Everything you've made significant about perceiving that emotion, so that you had to take it on, will you destroy and un-create all that please, and release it from your body?

One of the things that Gary and I have recently discovered is that when you perceive something, you then create a belief that that's the way it is. Let's say somebody wants to go out with you and you perceive it. You perceive their point of view, but rather than identifying it as their point of view, you have a belief about it. You may start to believe that you want to go out with them. If you perceive your mom doing a lot of sadness or your dad doing a lot of anger, you may end up believing life is full of sadness and anger. You have a perception of anger, and because of your perception, you create a belief that anger is the way life is, or sadness is the way life is.

How many things have you perceived about your Mom and Dad, which you turned into beliefs, and have been unable to let go of because you decided that's the way life is? Will you destroy and un-create all those, please?

When you make something significant, you create it locking in to the body. That emotion or that feeling or that thought locks into something called the focal point in the body. It becomes a focal point for the attraction of more of that. It's part of what locks the body up. When you intersect a cell with a thought, feeling or emotion, it starts to create a shift the in the structure of the cell, and it becomes more elliptical in shape. Scientists now believe that is the beginning of disease.

Don't make emotion, thoughts or feelings significant. They're just energy. The same goes for so-called traumatic events. If we wish to help people release the energy from abuse and trauma that has been locked up in their bodies, we are much more effective when we don't make those events significant, and we simply follow the energy.

Abuse

I suffered what some people might call pretty horrendous abuse when I was a kid. But even while I was experiencing it, I knew I would survive it just fine. Otherwise I wouldn't have chosen it. The idea that we chose to be abused may seem farfetched—but it comes up repeatedly with the people we work with who have been abused.

When I was doing Access processing to find out why I had experienced this abuse, I suddenly became aware that at the time I was being abused, I knew that if I allowed the abuse to occur, I would end the cycle of abuse with the person who was abusing me. It was something I chose. I knew that person would never be able to abuse anyone else again. So I allowed it to occur.

This is not an uncommon experience. Many people we have worked with have discovered that the abuse they experienced was something they chose. We worked with a lady who had been in therapy for years trying to handle her abuse issues. In her Access session, since nothing was clearing, she was asked, "Did you choose to be abused?"

She astonished herself with her answer. She said, "Yes, I chose it so I could get even with that fucker."

In an earlier lifetime, she had decided she would get back at the person who was abusing her no matter what it took. When the abuse occurred this lifetime, she was nine years old and he was 16. He had been the favored son in his family, but when she told what he had done, he was completely ostracized from his family, and to this day, he's a drunk on the street.

She successfully got back at him: She had decided that she would get him, and she did. Recognizing her decision about the abuse changed her life in the most amazing way. She went from being a victim to having a life.

I know this may come across as a weird point of view, and yet for me, the only thing that created freedom from the abuse I suffered was seeing that I had actually chosen it. Prior to understanding that, I had seen myself as a victim. I thought that was the reality. But I wasn't a victim—and seeing the truth of that freed me. I'm not saying this is true for everyone—but if you have abuse issues and you are not getting clarity from the therapy you're doing now, there are different possibilities you might want to look into. If you're getting really pissed off as you're reading this, it's probably true for you, too, and you haven't been willing to acknowledge it.

Releasing the energy of abuse

In Access we have some wonderful methods for allowing the body to return to a state of peace after clearing the issues of abuse. One of the techniques we use is called an Abuse Hold; it's a gentle and nurturing way of holding a person's body that allows the abuse that's been locked into the body to leach out.

I was using the Abuse Hold with a man who had been seriously sexually and physically abused, and who had previously done a lot of emotional release work. As I held him and the energy of the abuse began flowing out of his body, he started screaming an emotional release scream that he had been taught to do, and I was fascinated to observe that the energy, which had been releasing, stopped moving. He may have gotten release from the abuse on an emotional level, but his body did not get relief on a physical level.

Unfortunately, most emotional release work is not about following the person's energy. It tries to provide release, but it uses force generated outward by the person and can actually stop the energy from flowing. Release work has to be done from a place of beingness, not force and effort, and it's rare to find someone who understands that.

Affirmations

Affirmations can also stop the flow of energy, because with affirmations, you are attempting to create something that you don't believe actually exists. That's what affirmations are for. I believe I'm a piece of shit, so I'm going to say I smell like a rose. And what gets activated every time I say, I smell like a rose? I smell like shit. I smell like a rose—I smell like shit. The negative point of view is always lurking in the background, ready to be activated.

Most affirmations don't work because you're trying to use a polarity (I smell like a rose) to overcome a polarized point of view (I smell like shit). Polarity, no matter what form of it you're using, locks you into more polarity. Eventually the two polarities (shit and roses) have to come and meet each other. That's why the only source, the only solution, is consciousness. In consciousness you're not aligning and agreeing with smelling like shit, nor are you aligning and agreeing with smelling like a rose. Roses and shit are just an interesting point of view. That's consciousness.

What would happen if everything you experienced with your body was just an interesting point of view? What if you didn't resist and react against things? What would it be like if you didn't make energy significant, but simply followed it and allowed it to release?

THE POWER IN CARING

There's a huge amount of power in true caring. Most people, however, don't acknowledge—or even have a clue—about how much they actually care. In Access classes, we do an exercise that makes this real to people.

You can do it right now: Think of something or someone you have been upset with in the past week or so. Now, take all the feelings you have about that upset and make them infinite. Make them as big as the universe. Make them bigger than the universe. Not eternal, but infinite. You can imagine sticking the needle of a giant air pump into the middle of your upset, and then blowing it up so it's bigger than the universe, but making something bigger than the universe is not really something you have to think about or do. It's just an awareness, and it usually happens as soon as you're asked to do it.

What happens to those feelings of being upset when you make them infinite? Do they get fuller and more substantial? Do they have a greater sense of reality? Or do they fade away and disappear? If they fade away, which is what I suspect they will do, then they're a lie. The feeling and upset might be something you think are true, but they really aren't. You've bought something that's not true.

Now think about somebody you care about. Make that feeling infinite, bigger than the universe. Does it become more substantial or less substantial? More substantial? Isn't that interesting? When you think about how much you care for someone, and you make it infinite, bigger than the universe, you see it's even bigger than you're willing to admit to yourself.

When you take the caring that you have, and you make it infinite, it becomes fuller and more present. It occupies more space than the upset did. You realize that you care more than you acknowledge. You may say, "Yeah, yeah, I care," but when you fill it out and make it substantial, you can see how very much you care. It's almost as if we are afraid to care that much.

When you expand caring and make it infinite, your body begins to feel lighter and more peaceful. This is because you're acknowledging the caring that you as a being truly are. You don't have to do or be anything else. The only thing you have to do is stop hiding it and start acknowledging it. You have the caring and you are the caring. It's your power. You are the power.

Most of us only care for ourselves a tiny amount

Even with this infinite caring that we have and are, most of us only care for ourselves a tiny amount. This is all the caring we'll allow ourselves to have. Of the caring that's available, how much will we give to other people? Huge amounts. We'll do anything we can to make their lives easier, right? We'll do anything we can to get their bodies out of pain. We don't want to see the people we care about hurting. Will we do the same for ourselves and our bodies? No. What is that about? there Is a huge Power in caring for yourself

As a kid, were you taught to cry for what you wanted? Did you learn when you were a baby that crying was a perfect way to dominate, manipulate and control everybody? And as you got older, you realized, Oh, if I cry at the appropriate time, if I whine and act powerless, Mom and Dad will give me something. You learned that you could get others to care for you by acting powerless. What you weren't taught is that there is a huge power in caring for yourself.

In the family I grew up in, it was a sacrilege to care for yourself. "Hello? What do you mean you're not putting me first?" was the family's point of view. My dad was upset when I would do something for me. In fact, he still is. It's important to realize that most of the people you grew up around are either human—or humanoids desperately seeking to be human. Their points of view will always limit you. They desire no one to go beyond where they are. They desire no one to expand beyond them. People functioning from that human place feel a lot better when they are not challenged and nothing changes. They hate change, and discourage others from caring for themselves or doing anything that might cause them to change or grow.

You might have decided that caring for yourself and your body is selfishness and that it's not right to care for yourself. You might think that since other people are not caring for themselves, that you should follow their example and not care for yourself. You might have decided, I won't care for myself to the same degree they don't care for themselves. But this perpetuates an un-pretty reality in which people see that you're as limited as they are, rather than seeing that since you're more—they can be more, too.

SEXUALNESS

Have you ever had a really good massage from someone who really cared about your body? Most massage therapists do a massage by the numbers routine. These are definitely not nurturing and healing massages. They say, I do three strokes here and three strokes here and I make sure to cover up the private parts because I don't want to be sued. I don't want anybody to think I ever wanted to have sex in my life because they'd sue me if they knew I ever thought the body was beautiful, God forbid. Just about every massage therapist in the country is worried about being sued, and has totally cut off his or her sexualness. They even cut off their love of bodies, which is the thing that got them started in this profession in the first place.

I used to do massage when I was working my way through school. I used to massage people and I would cover up their bodies just like I was supposed to, but I would see how beautiful their bodies were and I'd get turned on while I was doing the massage. Would I think we were going to have sex? No. But I'd allow my sexualness to totally be there. Always.

People have told me years later, "I've had massages from twenty different people, and without a doubt, you gave me the best massage I ever had."

What was the ingredient in my massages that nobody else had? It was sexualness. Sexualness is the honoring, the nurturing, the acknowledging, the caring and the healing of the universe. It's the expansiveness, the creativity, and the gratitude. All of those elements are embodied in sexualness.

Because I would allow my sexualness to be there, my massage clients would tell me I gave them the most incredible massages they'd ever had.

Embodying the sexualness of you

One of the essential characteristics of embodiment is being the sexualness you truly are. Embodying the sexualness of you allows everything else in your life to show up.

One of the ways we easily experience our sexualness is when we're out in nature. We're out there in the fresh air and sunlight with no other people around. We receive energy from the plants and animals and the Earth and everything else. We don't cut anything off. Doing this energizes the body, and if we're willing to truly receive the energy that's there, we might start to feel our body vibrate or become more alive. The same thing can happen when we go into the ocean, if we're willing to perceive it and receive it. We're willing to be totally sexual with everything around us, we're in communion with everything. That is what the energy of sexualness feels like. We're in Oneness with everything around us. Do we put up barriers to receiving anything? No. Do we see a yellowed leaf and say, "What an ugly shade of yellow. I can't believe they left that yellow leaf here.

Can somebody come clean that up, please?" No, we don't judge anything. We don't have any reason to cut off our receiving.

When you're experiencing this energy in nature, do you feel less sexual—or more? More! I have a friend who used to say, "I don't know what it is, but when I go camping, I masturbate the whole time." You're out in nature, and there's no one around to turn you on, and you feel more sexual and turned-on than you do in the city, where you are surrounded by people. Isn't that interesting?

When you understand what your sexualness is, and you begin to embody it, you can bring the same turned-on feeling you experience in nature to your everyday life.

Are you vibrantly alive and willing to receive the energy of the universe?

Imagine one of those mornings when you wake up and you are on. You are alive. You feel great and you are ready to go. Hallelujah. How does it get any better than that? That's a lot of sexualness. That's the sexualness you truly have and are. No-sexualness is when you wake up on another morning and you say, Oh shit, I've got to get up. Oh please, let me hit the snooze button for another eight hours. In one mode, you're vibrantly alive and willing to receive the energy of the universe and in the other, you want to hit the snooze button and shut out the world. That's about as easy as it gets to recognize the difference.

When you leave your sexualness on, your body's willing to receive so much more. When you touch somebody else's body with your sexualness present, their body melts for you. You create a healing shift in their body just by touching it with total presence and total sexualness.

Are you willing to do that with your body and other people's bodies? A lot of people have made decisions and judgments about why it's bad to touch and be touched. Some people, especially young girls, are warned by their mothers against being expansive, open and friendly: Watch out, dear. Don't talk to them. If you talk to them like that you know what's going to happen? Really bad stuff. Some people are reluctant to touch other people's bodies with sexualness because they think sexualness is an invitation for copulation. It isn't. Sexualness is simply the honoring, the nurturing, the acknowledging, the caring and the healing of the universe. It's the expansiveness of the universe, the creativity, and the gratitude.

SEX, SEXUALNESS, SENSUALNESS, COPULATION & SEXUALITY

A lot of confusion gets created around the words sex, sexualness, sensuality, copulation and sexuality. Each one of those terms means a completely different thing, but they are all part of the greatness of embodiment.

Sex is when you're looking good, feeling good, and strutting your stuff. It's when you're wearing a sexy outfit and you know everybody's looking at you because you're feeling great and you're totally willing to receive their attention and admiration.

Sensualness has to do with all the pleasant sensations your body gets to experience. It's your body loving to be touched, delighting in the sensation of the sun on your skin and enjoying the feel of water as you swim through it. It's the touching and the sensations of the body. That's sensualness.

Copulation is the act of putting the bodies together. Notice that sex and copulation are not the same thing. We often use sex to mean the same thing as copulation, but this tends to confuse people by giving them one word that means something else. Copulation is simply putting the bodies together.

Sexuality is probably the most misidentified and misapplied word in this whole area. People think sexuality is about copulation and sex, but that's not what sexuality is. Sexuality is your definition of your sexual nature and it's always your judgment. An example of sexuality is: I'm a straight man or I'm a gay man. I'm a three-legged gay donkey may be an observation, but it's also sexuality. I'm a gay woman.

I'm a straight woman. I'm bisexual. I'm trisexual. I'll try any kind of sex there is. That last one is probably closer to not having sexuality, because there's no judgment in it. At any rate, sexuality is always a judgment. It cuts off what you can receive from others. Along with sexuality comes the force and judgment of cutting off some aspect of you in order to make your delineated sexuality work. Some degree of force is needed in order to make the judgment valid and to hold it in place and to keep the form, structure, and significance of it from being destroyed.

When I define myself as a straight male, am I willing to receive sexual energy or sexualness from gay males? No. Am I willing to receive sexual energy from straight males? No. Am I willing to receive sexual energy from gay women? No. The only place I'll allow myself to receive sexualness is with heterosexual women. Do you see a slight limitation in that?

And that's just talking about the two-leggeds. If I define myself as a straight male, am I able to receive energy from trees, plants, grass, air and water? The answer is no. When you define your sexuality, you cut off your ability and willingness to receive from anything that's not included in your judgment.

If I'm a gay woman, am I willing to receive energy from straight men? No. Gay men? No. Straight women? No. Isn't that interesting? If you're not willing to receive their energy, are you willing to receive their money? No. If you're not willing to receive their energy, and you're not willing to receive their money, you'll find you're not really willing to receive much of anything at all.

When you're functioning from true sexualness, you have no judgment of anyone or anything. You have no judgment of their bodies, and you have no judgment of your own. You may have a preference one way or the other. You may choose to copulate with people of the same sex or with the other sex, but you don't cut off the energy that you're willing to receive from anyone.

Gary and I were once teaching a woman how to attract the person into her life that she would like to be with. Gary said, "And if that person shows up in the same sex body as you ..."

And the woman hurriedly said, "I could never do that! I could never have sex with a woman!"

With that point of view, what do you think you project to your partner about having sex with you? If you can't consider the possibility of having sex with your own body, what do you think might be going on in the other person's head?

So, I invite you to destroy and uncreate all of those judgments you have of your body type or the other body type. Notice I don't say the opposite sex? I say the other sex. That's because the word opposite creates an opposition.

In true sexualness, you don't function from sexuality. I have broken these elements down so you don't misidentify and misapply them, because if you're misidentifying and misapplying them, you're continually buying a lie and there's no way to get freedom and joy around sexualness because you're always looking in the wrong place.

THE 1, 2, 3 OF SEX VS THE COMMUNION OF SEXUALNESS

Have you ever noticed how many judgments come up that keep you from having communion with your body? Most of us are not able to be present because we're continually judging. We have judgments of our bodies, judgments of our capacity, judgments of our abilities sexually: Am I doing the right thing? Am I touching him the right way? Am I making her feel good? Does he like this? Is my penis big enough? Is my vagina tight enough? Are my breasts big enough? Does he like the way my nipples look? Does she like my butt?

From my point of view, copulation should be a time when you and your partner are both totally present. You are expanding, having fun, experiencing intense energy and willing to touch, lick, kiss or suck any part of the other person's body. Afterwards your body feels great and your partner's body feels great.

Have you ever copulated like that with somebody?

Some people tell me that the first time they copulated with their partner it was like that—but then it changed.

What happened?

It's the 1, 2, 3 rule of relationship. The first time you copulate with somebody, it's for fun. The second time you copulate with them, you're in relationship. The third time you copulate with them, you're getting married. You think I'm full of shit, don't you?

Embodiment. The Manual You Should Have Been Given When You Were Born

The first time I heard Gary say this, I went into such resistance. I thought, "That's not true!" I figured I'd put it to the test.

I copulated with somebody and it was great and it was wonderful and she left happy and I left happy and wow, it was awesome and expansive and so much fun. I thought, "That was great. Let's try this again. I'm sure the next time will be even more fun."

It started out fun the second time and about midway through, something was going on; things started feeling a little heavy and twisted, but I didn't know why and couldn't figure it out. I thought, "Wow, this was so intensely sexual the first time, and now it's turning into ...." I tried to talk myself out of it, and wondered what was wrong with me, but there it was.

By the second time you're already thinking about what it would be like to be in relationship with the person and do they like the same color carpet you do, and do they like your towels, and will their cat pee on your head while you're sleeping. Your body is saying, "Stop it, please. You're killing me. Stop." But you've already decided, "No, this person is so great. We're going to be in a great relationship together." That's the second time you copulated. And you're already beginning to wonder if they'll call you in the morning and planning what piss-mark you're going to leave behind. Should you leave an earring—or a pair of undies—in the bed?

The third time the heaviness gets more intense. You're in the process of deciding whether you want to be with them forever. Your body is trying to tell you, "You are trapping us in this." Are you listening? No. Generally not. You're ignoring your body and cutting off its awareness.

Sometimes women tell me that they've functioned from an unspoken rule that they cannot copulate with someone just once. It wouldn't be right. If they did it just once, they'd be a slut; they'd be a whore. Guys know they're supposed to go out and have one night stands as often as they can to prove they're men. And women know that if they sleep with somebody just once, they're a slut. Huh? Is that real? Or is it something they created and inferred from the judgments and the trappings of this reality? What does that judgment have to do with how wonderfully nurturing it is to be in the presence of your beautiful body? And your body being in the presence of somebody else's beautiful body? What does any of that have to do with any of that?

Unfortunately, most people have judgments that when they copulate with somebody it's supposed to mean something. A lot of people think this—but what they don't know is that making copulation significant, or looking for the meaning in it, destroys the infinite possibilities that are available. When you decide, Oh I'm going to copulate with him, and it's going to be so much fun, and then we'll have a relationship, and then maybe he'll want to get married. And he'll buy me a house and a car, then we'll have children, and we'll live happily ever after, you've had it.

The way you know you have the 1, 2, 3 program going on in your universe is when you start wondering what they're doing, getting upset when they don't call, getting jealous of who they're spending time with and wanting them to make you more of a priority than the other people and things in their life. If you go to any of those places, you are already doing relationship, and are on your way to creating a marriage. And in the process, you end up not only destroying the sexualness that is there and available, you also cut off the receiving that your body could have and the joy, because copulation should be a joyful expression of life.

Do you have any part of the 1, 2, 3 program going on in your universe? Or do you feel free, if you see someone who looks like they're going to be fun and nurturing to your body, to get together and touch bodies? You might copulate and you might not, based on your mutual choice and what's most expansive in the moment. You'd have a great time and at the end would give them a kiss on the cheek and say, "Thank you so much," and never have to have it again. Each time would be so awesome and wonderful that you would have tremendous gratitude for the other person and for you. It would be a completion or a fulfillment unto itself. Are you willing to have that as your reality?

I'm not advocating that everyone go out and do bed-hopping as their method of creating their life; what I'm saying is whatever you choose to do, it should be from a place of joy. It should always be a choice. And it should always be with the awareness of what you're creating in your universe and in the universe of the person you are copulating with.

I'm not saying, "Don't have sex" or "Do have sex."

But please, have a lot of sex.

ORGASM

(If you're expecting this to be endorsed by the Pope, don't read it.)

Let's talk about orgasm. Orgasmic energy is creative energy. It's literally the energy of creation. When you have that energy running through your body all the time, you're always on. And when you're burning with that intensity, it allows you to confront anything. Have you ever noticed that when you're running on low intensity, no orgasm energy, you can more easily buy into a limited human reality?

If you'd like to experience the greatness of embodiment, my suggestion is to touch your body and masturbate more. I suggest this to people and tell them, "If you think I'm full of shit, and you try it anyway and decide I'm not full of shit, you owe me a dollar," and there are a few daring souls who actually try it. Every single one of them who has done it more than once has come to me and said, "I thought you were full of shit. Here's a buck. I thought you were full of shit, but oh my God. Oh my God! Oh my God! Hallelujah!" Please don't just masturbate once a day. Do it more than once. More than once a day is truly what your body is asking for.

How many orgasms would your body like to have in a day?

In a recent workshop on Embodiment, I asked participants, "How many orgasms—if you were to have no barriers, no considerations, no judgments, no past and no history—how many orgasms would your body like to have in a day?" Some people had a hard time answering. Some went outside the realm of what they would actually allow themselves to receive. I told them it was okay if their answer went beyond the realm of the possible and the attainable. Some people said three, some said seven or eight, some said 12 or 15, some said 47 or 55, and one person said unlimited.

When I asked my body this question about a year ago, my body's answer was eight. I thought, That's impossible! How's that going to happen?

Notice that first I said, "That's impossible," which is an answer—and then I asked a question, "How's that going to happen?" Then I said, "Wait a minute, what if that weren't impossible?

I revoked, recanted, rescinded, reclaimed, renounced, destroyed and un-created every judgment and every decision that it was impossible. Eight orgasms? How's that going to happen? Well, it hasn't quite happened—yet. But it has made me aware that my body desires a lot more than I was willing to acknowledge. I thought once a day was great, but my body was saying, "You know, we could probably easily do about three a day," and I said, "Okay cool."

Since I've done that, my body's had so much more energy. Where do I find the time? I don't know. We just seem to make the time for things that are important. By the way, the muscle tone has increased, too. And not just in the right arm, despite what you might be thinking.

There's a false idea that orgasm is a completion

Orgasm feeds your body energetically. There's a false idea that orgasm is a completion. It's one of the biggest lies that has been perpetuated in the sexual arena. It's a lie specifically designed to make sure you never have an orgasmic reality. Orgasm isn't the completion of sex; it should be the state of your life.

You ought to be able to be orgasmic and continue to be orgasmic all through your life. You shouldn't have to shift or change. You should actually be able to have orgasm after orgasm after orgasm, but that's a story for another time.

Have you ever had an orgasm and it kept happening, you just laughed and laughed and laughed? This is what's possible. Start on your own if you want to, and ideally when you have a partner, he or she will be as exploratory and into having fun as you are. Hopefully he or she will have such gratitude for your body and be in such joy and pleasure of it that sex becomes an expansive activity that allows you the freedom to explore every possibility that presents itself.

When we conduct our classes and workshops, we try to be open to the energy that comes up and follow it. We notice which direction the energy goes and we follow it. This leads to a lot of transformation for the people who are participating. From almost out of left field something comes up that ties together—and clears out—everything we were working on. What if sex were like that? What if you followed the energy and were open to what came up? Most people do sex by the numbers. They say, One, I'm going to touch my partner this way; two, this way; three, this way. Now I'm going to repeat that four times. Okay, now I'm moving down here. Now I'm going to do this. Twenty-eight, 29, 30. What happened? I didn't get the response I was looking for. Thirty-nine, 40, 41, 42.

Why do people do sex by numbers? Is it because they're stupid and incompetent? No. It's because nobody's been taught. Nobody's been shown what true sexualness is.

Nobody's been shown what the greatness of copulation can be. Nobody's been shown how expansive it truly can be.

There's a different sexual possibility available than anything you've considered. You may have experienced snippets of what's possible, or you may have experienced large parts of what's possible. Sex should be fun. It should be caring and nurturing to your body all the way through. It should leave you and your partner with smiles on your faces and your bodies glowing.

Now, just for the fun of it, let's try something to see how your body feels. Remember what the energy of orgasm was like even if it's been 150 years since you had one. Now, take that energy and pull it up through your feet through your body and out the top of your head. How does your body feel? Better? More alive? Just keep doing that all day long. You wouldn't do it all day long for what reason?

EVERYTHING IN YOUR LIFE SHOULD BE AN ORGASMIC EXPERIENCE

Everything in your life should be an orgasmic experience. Your body loves it when you function from orgasmic energy. You can experience this when you eat. As you sit down at the table, create a little bubble around you and your body for the moment, and ask your body what it desires to eat. It's just you and your body.

Be aware that bodies are always picking up information from other people's bodies. Create a little bubble around your body so you know it's your body you're talking to and you don't unintentionally pick up what other people's bodies are asking for. Then ask your body, "What would you like to eat?" Look down at the menu and something will catch your eye, and you might say, But I don't like that. Check it out with your body. Ask, "Would you like that?" and your body will say yes or no.

It may take a while to get it right. You may order a few shitty meals at first. That's okay. This is how to start being in communion with your body and knowing what it's asking for. When you ask, don't be surprised if it says soup or salad, a side order or sunlight. Sunlight and water and sex. Bodies like those.

When your food arrives, put one bite in your mouth, and before you chew it, notice how it affects every taste bud on your tongue. What happens when you chew it? When you swallow? Eat the first three bites of each thing on your plate in total awareness. You may find that three bites of each thing satisfy your body, and if you do, that's fine. When it stops tasting absolutely wonderful and it starts tasting like cardboard, your body is done. It's had enough.

Most of us tend not to have much of a sense of our bodies. Have you noticed that? You ask, What does my body desire? and you don't have a friggin' clue what it's asking of you or what it's requiring or what would make it feel good. Somewhere in the scheme of things we gave that awareness up. If you want to start enjoying life as an orgasmic experience, you need to develop your awareness of your body.

CONVERSATIONS WITH BOD. 10 THINGS YOUR BODY WOULD TELL YOU IF ONLY YOU'D LISTEN

There are ten things your body is requesting of you.

1. Do one thing a day to nurture, acknowledge and appreciate me

The first thing your body is saying is: "Do one thing a day to nurture, acknowledge and appreciate me."

How many days do you manage to nurture, acknowledge and appreciate your body? Every day? About three out of seven? About one out of 800? Your body would like you to acknowledge it and nurture it on a daily basis.

One lady we worked with asked her body, "Okay body, how would you like for me to nurture you and acknowledge you?"

Her body said, "I'd like to be powdered."

She said, "Powdered?"

"Yeah, powdered," it said. "Like your mom used to do." Her mother used to powder her body after her bath every night, and it was an experience of great nurturing for her. That's what her body asked for. She began to powder it every night after her bath, and she lost 25 pounds within a matter of weeks. The weight literally dropped off because she was nurturing her body in the way it wished to be nurtured.

Touching your body is a great way to communicate with it, and to nurture, acknowledge and appreciate it. When you wake up in the morning, gently touch or stroke your body for three minutes. Run your hands over your arms, over your legs, over your feet, over your stomach, over your chest, over your neck, over your face. When you touch your body, touch it as if it belongs to somebody that you care for very much. Feel your body. Let it feel you. Receive from it, and let it receive from you. Bodies love to be touched sensually. Sensuality is one of their greatest joys. They love to receive touch from a caring place with total sexualness.

Do you want a face-lift? Would you like to erase wrinkles and lines and firm up the skin on your face? When you wake up tomorrow morning, put your hands on your face for five minutes—or for two minutes. Simply put your hands on your face and connect with your body.

What you body actually wants you to do is to put your hands on your face for two minutes, then touch the rest of your body, and then masturbate. Who the hell cares if you're late for whatever it is, if that's what you're doing?

2. Stop judging me

I'm speaking for your body, okay? I'm sorry, but the second thing your body is saying is: "Stop fucking judging me." Judging your body is not the way to change it. Instead, acknowledge it and then ask it what it would take for it to change.

Your body is as conscious as you are, maybe even more so, because it's willing to be. It's like an animal. Animals are conscious, simply because they don't cut off their awareness with judgments like we do.

If you judge your body, is that going to help it shift and change? Absolutely not. Instead, what if you lived in the question, and asked it, "Body, what would it take for this to change?" You might be surprised by what happens. Just ask it, "Hey body, what would it take for ____ to show up? What would it take to look this way?" If you ask your body a question, you'll get what you're looking for from it.

Of course, then you have to listen to what it says!

When you look in the mirror in the morning, make a conscious choice to stop the litany of judgment that you start with each and every day. Your body is saying, "Instead of judging me, thank me and tell me how grateful you are for me." Do you ever do that? Do you ever say, "Body, thank you so much. You have put up with so much crap and so much judgment. You put up with so much junk that I've thrown your way. Thank you. Thanks for allowing me to continue to be in communion with you and connected to you, because if I were you, I would've kicked my ass a long time ago."

Instead of judging the parts that are too big, the parts that are too small, the parts that are too lumpy, or whatever the judgment happens to be, touch those parts of your body and say, "Thank you so much for being here. Thanks for being a part of my body. Thanks for being my shoulder."

3. I was created to have fun

The third thing your body is saying to you is: "I was created to have fun."

I have a startling question to ask you: What if the sole purpose of life was to have fun? Some people say life is supposed to be fun for kids, but not for adults. They think adults have heavy and serious responsibilities, so they can't have fun, and a lot of people have ended up buying this point of view.

But let's look at it: Is having responsibility really heavy and serious? Is that view of responsibility a truth—or is it a myth?

There's a simple little test you can use to determine the truth of things: The truth always makes you feel lighter. A lie always makes you feel heavier. If something makes you feel heavy, it's a lie for you, whether or not it is for anybody else.

What does responsibility feel like for you? Is it light, happy, joyous, expansive and easy? Or is it heavy, heavy, heavy? For me, responsibility is a myth. I can take care of all kinds of things in life and have a great time. What about you? Why don't you destroy the myth of responsibility as obligation and burden and all the seriousness and heaviness that entails?

So, let's return to fun. What if the sole purpose of life were to have fun? Would that change the way you do things? For your body, it's fun to feel the sun on its skin. It's fun to be touched. It's fun to walk with its feet in the grass, its feet on the sand, its feet in the water. It's fun to feel a new texture. It's fun to have really great sheets and a feather bed with down comforter. It's fun to have soft clothing.

What if you started to have fun right now?

4. Ask me about me

The fourth thing your body is saying is: "Ask me about me. Don't do things that involve me without asking me how I feel about them. Don't do anything to me without asking me first. That's simple enough, right? Don't shove hummus up my nose because someone tells you it will make us feel sexy and lose weight."

How much fad crap have you done to your body because somebody said it would create a result? Excuse me. Yes, what you need to do is eat the intestines of this poisonous spider because what it will do is make you lose your cellulite. Huh?

I've got an easy answer for all of those fad body solutions: Ask your body. Stop judging and ask your body. Your body has all the answers if you'll start asking.

5. Ask me what it would take to get me to look the way you want me to

Point five has to do with how the body looks. Your body is saying: "If you'll just ask what it would take to get me to look the way you want me to, I'll be happy to comply. I'll let you know exactly what it would take, but you never ask and take the time to listen and then do what I request."

If you want to get your body to look a certain way, acknowledge the greatness of it as it is, and then ask it what it would take to shift something you want to change. "Body, What would it take to shift this and make this bigger and this smaller?" If you do this, you'll have an awareness of what it will take.

My body's been asking for something like Pilates for a long time. Have I been listening? Hell no. My excuse has been that I travel all the time, but the other day I found Pilates on DVD that I can use anywhere. My body's saying, "Start doing the DVD." Okay. Sorry. I did about ten pushups this morning before I had to get in the shower and get ready and eat my Corn Pops, and my body was saying, "Thank you."

I asked, "Is that enough?"

It said, "Yeah, that will be fine."

When you're in communion with your body, and when you're willing to acknowledge what it tells you, your body will create miracles from tiny amounts of input. We tend to believe in the human reality that it takes huge amounts of force to create a shift in your body: You have to work out an hour a day six times a week. You have to do cardio. You have to do some kind of strength training exercise. You have to eat properly. You have to stretch. You have to eat right for your blood type.

Do you ever get confused by all the information out there about what's supposed to make a body work well, feel good and look good? I've got a solution for you. Ask your body what will be good for it. It will deny and throw out 99.9 percent of all the things you suggest, and there will be one thing that will actually work. But you have to ask.

Some people have given up and believe they can't get the results they want with their bodies. They've tried a million things without ever once asking their bodies what would work. When your body does something unusual, like taking up more space or decreasing in size, you can ask it, "Okay body, what awareness are you sharing with me here? What awareness is this that I'm not willing to have?" Say your body suddenly shrinks. Ask, "Okay body, what's going on? What's really happening here that I'm not willing to acknowledge?" It will tell you.

Your body is a sensory organ and it picks up information of all kinds. If you experience pain or discomfort, it may not really be your body's pain; it may be an awareness it has. You can ask it, "What awareness are you sharing with me that I'm not willing to receive?"

It may take a little while. You might not get the answer immediately, but as you increase your awareness, your body will show you what's going on. It's happened to me a number of times. Remember that any time you're asking your body a question about what will work for it, the answer is probably not going to be verbal; it will probably be an energy. And it may not happen immediately. The lady who found the diet that was correct for her body by overhearing some people talk about it, had to wait a while until she was in the right place to hear the information she needed.

Know that when you ask the question, your body will do everything it can to get you where it needs to be for you to hear the right information. Everything that doesn't allow you to be willing to hear that information, will you now destroy and un-create all that, please.

The more aware you become, and the more willing you are to let go of your fixed points of view, the more flexible your body becomes, and the faster things can change. Not long ago, Gary and I were playing Frisbee in the park across from our house. I was throwing the Frisbee and he was running, and trying to jump like an old man. He's 62, but he looks 45, and he's the most flexible person I've ever seen. But he could not run to save his life and when he went to jump it was, "Oh please don't do that again."

Finally I said, "Wait a minute. What the fuck are you doing?"

He said, "What do you mean?"

I said, "You are one of the most flexible people I've ever known in my life. You'll let go of a point of view faster than anyone I've ever seen. You'll completely change your point of view on something when you get new information, just like that. Why are you acting like an inflexible, old fucking man?"

He said, "Oh, good point," and he instantaneously stopped moving like an inflexible old man. He threw the Frisbee back to me. I caught it. I threw it to him again and he was running like a 30-year old instead of a 70-year old. That's how quickly your body can change if you're willing to have flexibility with your beingness also.

6. I'm the one eating

Point six has to do with eating. Your body is saying, "I'm the one eating, idiot. You are not."

Okay, I just added idiot. Your body didn't really say that. But it did say, "When it comes time to eat, ask me what I'd like."

My body changes every day. It likes meat some days, vegetables some days, fruit some days, and just dessert some days.

Your body is saying, "You assume that because you like green beans, I should like green beans. I say again, I'm the one eating. Ask me what I'd like to eat."

There is a kid in Houston who is about 11 or 12, and he and his mom have been doing Access, and they learned about asking the body what it wants to eat. One day, the kid said, "Mom, my body wants ice cream for breakfast."

His mom asked, "Does your body really want that?"

He said, "Yes, it does."

She said, "Okay," and let him have ice cream.

Then a little later on he said, "Mom, I'm hungry again."

She said, "What does your body want?"

He said, "Ice cream."

She said, "Okay," and let him have ice cream five times that day.

The sixth time he said he was hungry, his mom asked, "What does your body want?"

Again he said, "Ice cream," because he was testing her. He was seeing if she would go for it.

She let him have it again and he threw up.

So, be careful how you try to dominate, manipulate and control your body because it may not work.

7. Ask me what movement I would like to do

Point seven has to do with moving your body. Instead of asking your body what exercise it would like, ask it what movement it would like to do. What movement. It might be dancing, it might be Pilates. Just ask. It might be riding, cycling, running, roller-blading, running on the beach, doing push-ups, yoga, or Hula hoops. It might want to do something completely different every single day. Maybe your body wants to do gymnastics. One of the things my body likes to do is shoot arrows. It loves shooting arrows because it's an exercise in beingness as well as a little bit of movement. But the point is: Ask your body what movement it would like to do, and it will let you know.

When I started doing Access about five years ago, my body was like a bodybuilder's. It was all stiff and tight. I walked like a mechanical man. Now I can be present in my body and move it and it moves with me and we're together. When you're truly in communion with your body, moving it is a joy and a pleasure. Have you ever watched a cat walk? Have you noticed how they use every muscle in their bodies when they move? They never turn off their sexualness.

Have you noticed that the only cats that ever get sick and stiff are the cats that take on their owners' disease, problems, and points of view? When cats in the wild start to get sick and stiff, they go off and die. They say, "I'm done. 'Bye." Cats have a really interesting point of view. So do dogs, wolves, birds and every other animal that's out in the wild and functioning from choice. What do they do when their bodies start falling apart? They lie down and die. For them, if it ain't fun being here, they ain't gonna do it. "If I'm not hopping around, having sex, living in the sun, flying, walking, running, using every muscle in my body, and enjoying it, it's bye-bye. That was fun. I'm going to go and get another body." They don't attach significance to their bodies or consider that keeping them alive is more important than taking joy in them.

The point here is that bodies love to move. Ask your body what movement it would like to do. It will let you know.

8. Don't buy the latest fad

Point eight has to do with fads. Your body says, "Don't buy the latest fad as to what will finally change me. I don't need to be changed as much as I need to be listened to." Your body would just like you to listen to it and it will change anything you want. It's really simple.

9. Ask, "Where does this come from?"

Point nine has to do with how to handle pains, discomforts and hunger. Instead of reactively responding to these when you feel them, your body wants you to ask, "Where does this come from?" Every time you experience, pain, discomfort and hunger, simply ask the question: Where does this come from?

Ninety-eight percent of the thoughts, feelings and emotions you experience aren't yours. And somewhere between 50 percent to 90 percent of the pain and suffering you experience in your body isn't yours. Never was.

If you ask, Where does this come from? and it lightens up, it's not yours. Just return it to sender.

Gary worked with a woman who would eat three or four doughnuts every day at work. She wanted to change that behavior, so every time she thought she had to have a doughnut, she'd ask, "Who does this belong to?" or "Where does this come from?" She realized she was eating doughnuts for the people she worked with, who wanted doughnuts and were resisting them. She discovered that she wasn't really hungry for doughnuts at all, and she lost 25 pounds in four weeks. True story.

10. I'm a body and you're an infinite being

Point number ten: Your body is saying, "Hey, I'm a body. You're an infinite being. You're not inside of me. I am inside of you. Because you're infinite, which is really, really, really big, you're too immense to fit inside of me. Rather, I exist inside of you, but that doesn't mean we shouldn't have a connection and a communion, right?"

Those are the ten things your body wants from you. Simple, right? Light and easy. It's quite different from the sledgehammer approach, which takes a lot of pain and suffering. Embodiment doesn't require pain and suffering. Not if you're in communion. A feather touch creates a huge result. But you have to listen to the ten things your body is saying.

HAVE A LITTLE GRATITUDE

Before I started Access, I used to work out five to six times a week for at least an hour at a time. I had to do that and I had to eat like a friggin'—I'd say like a horse—except they don't eat enough for what I was eating. I weighed probably 20 pounds more than I weigh now. I would go to Carl's Jr. and I'd order three chicken sandwiches and a hamburger and a large fries and a large refillable Coke and I would eat it all. Super-size me. It was a huge amount of food and that's what I thought my body required.

I was tired all the time. How long would it take your body to digest that much food? All friggin' day, except I did it three times a day. I would eat eight eggs in the morning—four whole eggs and four egg whites with cheese or ham, plus four pieces of toast. At lunchtime, I'd have all those sandwiches. And then at dinner I'd have at least two huge platefuls of rice and curry or pork chops or whatever it happened to be. My body felt like shit.

The weird part is that's what I thought I had to do to feel good, and to keep my body looking good. It required huge amounts of working out and force to do that. Now I work out maybe once every couple of weeks. I jog a few times a week. If I'm at home, I'll cycle or ride my horse. That's about it, and my body feels so much better.

Are there shifts I keep asking my body to make? Yes. Are there some it hasn't made yet that I keep asking for? Yes. Are there some days that I get up and judge my body? Yes. Does my body feel good on those days? No. But it does feel great when I get up and say from a place of gratitude, "You know what, body? You're so good to me. Thank you so much." My body starts feeling great and it starts creating itself as what I would like to see.

Are you willing to have gratitude for your body? I can hear your body thanking me for telling you this. It's saying, "I've been doing such a good job!"

Our bodies are doing a damn good job for us, and it's amazing that they're still here and haven't kicked our asses out. It is absolutely amazing that your body does what it does with what you've given it until now. But look at it. If it's been able to do what it's been able to do with what you've saddled it with, imagine what it can do from this point forward, with your acknowledgment, gratitude and communication. It's only going to get better. Just keep asking: How does it get any better than this? What are the infinite possibilities?

Some people I talk with are interested in embodiment in terms of cool feats and tricks they can perform. I tell them that cool feats are available, but you can't go from the human embodiment of judgment and limitation, which doesn't acknowledge the body, the caring or the sexualness of you, to creating three arms and four legs instantaneously. You have to unlock the limitations and judgments before you can do tricks. You've got to be in communion with your body before you can possibly create any other result with it.

You may have some areas where you're thinking, I'd like a better this. I'd like a better that. That's okay. The way to approach these ideas of bettering your body is through the space of infinite caring and gratitude. Instead of looking at your body and saying, I'd like a better this or that, begin with total gratitude: "Wow, body, you're so fucking cool. Thank you!" Be grateful that it's willing to allow you to exist as the space between its molecules.

How much gratitude are you willing to have for your body right now? Gratitude is, I believe, what love was supposed to be. Express your gratitude to your body: "Thank you, body. Thank you for moving me from here to there. Thank you for having such a wonderful night's sleep. Thanks for allowing me to feel this wonderful sensation on our skin. Thank you for allowing me to experience this orgasmic taste."

Come out of judgment of yourself for not being perfect

Embodiment starts with being in communion with your body, and the primary elements of that are gratitude, sexualness and a willingness to be in communion. You're willing to receive your body exactly as it is. You have no judgment. If you find you have a judgment, destroy and un-create it. Send it back to the nasty turkey that gave it to you in the first place.

Having gratitude allows you to receive, and the receiving allows you to have gratitude. It goes both ways. And this will allow you to experience the greatness of embodment, which includes total sexualness, total caring, total healing, total nurturing, total expansiveness and total joy.

Those are the possibilities that are available. Please be kind to yourself. Be kind to your body. Be extremely kind to you as you continue to become more aware of your body. You will have great changes and great transformations and shifts and the whole thing doesn't occur in two days. You've been creating limitations for four trillion years or so. Sometimes it takes a little longer than two days to get rid of some of them, so don't judge yourself for your limitations. That's my request of you. Please come out of judgement of you for not being perfect. Because, truly, you are.

A NOTE TO READERS

Access is an energy transformation program which links seasoned wisdom, ancient knowledge and channeled energies with highly contemporary motivational tools. Its purpose is to set you free by giving you access to your truest, highest self.

The information, tools and techniques presented in this book are just a small taste of what Access has to offer. There is a whole universe of Access processes and classes.

If there are places where you can't get things in your life to work the way you know they ought to you might be interested in attending an Access class or workshop or locating an Access facilitator, who can work with you to give you greater clarity about issues you can't overcome. Access processes are done with a trained facilitator, and are based on the energy of you and the person you're working with.

www.accessconsciousness.com

OTHER ACCESS BOOKS

Conscious Parents Conscious Kids
This book is a collection of narratives from children immersed in living with conscious awareness.

Money is Not the Problem, You Are.
Offering out-of-the-box concepts with money. Its not about money. It never is. Its about what you're willing to receive.

Talk To The Animals
Did you know that every animal, every plant, every structure on this planet has consciousness and desires to gift to you?

Embodiment: The Manual You Should Have Been Given When You Were Born
Introducing you to the awareness that there really is a different choice.

Sex Is Not a Four Letter Word but Relationship Often Times Is
Funny, frank, and delightfully irreverent, this book offers readers an entirely fresh view of how to create great intimacy and exceptional sex.

Magic. You are it. Be it
Magic is about the fun of having the things you desire. The real magic is the ability to have the joy that life can be.

ACCESS SEMINARS, WORKSHOPS & CLASSES

If you liked what you read in this book and are interested in attending Access seminars, workshops or classes, then for a very different point of view, read-on and sample a taste of what is available.

www.AccessConsciousness.com

ACCESS BARS CLASS

One-Day

Bars is one of the foundational tools of Access. You will learn a hands-on energetic process, which you will gift and receive during the class. The bars process has created massive amounts of ease and change for people all over the world. The bars consist of 32 points on the head which hold the electrical energetic charge of the thoughts, ideas, beliefs, decisions, and emotions that you have stored in any lifetime about: Healing, Body, Time, Hopes, Control, Awareness, Creativity, Power, Aging, Sex, Money, and so forth. The bars are activated by a light touch, allowing energy to flow. This creates greater ease in your body and opens new possibilities, freeing the "stuck" areas of your life and allowing you to choose in the present rather than from the past. Every time you gift a bars session to someone, you receive the benefits as well. This class is wonderful for any bodywork practitioners, as well as for people who have always wanted to learn a dynamic energetic process. It is also a way for you to experience receiving, rather than the doing, doing, doing that people are always taught.

Prerequisites: None

www.AccessConsciousness.com

ACCESS FOUNDATION CLASS

Two-Day

This class invites you to look at where you reside in the "I have no choice" universe- to change it! You will gain clarity on how you have used reason, justification, beliefs, and judgments to create your reality, as well as awareness of the energetic structures that are obstructing your ability to change. The clearings you receive from this class will allow you to claim, own, and acknowledge your potency to transform anything that isn't working for you. You will receive tools to recognize truth and lies, to utilize language and energy to generate your life, as well as learning a dynamic hands-on process to heal cellular memory in bodies.

Prerequisites: Bars Class

www.AccessConsciousness.com

ACCESS LEVEL ONE CLASS

Two-Day

This class expands on the possibilities opened in the Foundation class and covers areas of sexualness, money, abundance, and the five elements of intimacy. The clearings allow you to eliminate limitations and distractors, as well as to gain clarity about some of the greatest lies of this reality. You can generate relationships in which you are honored. You may receive greater awareness of infinite beingness and infinite choice, so you can perceive, know, be, and receive with ease. You will also learn another amazing, hands-on body process called MTVSS.

Prerequisites: Bars & Foundation Class

www.AccessConsciousness.com

ACCESS LEVEL 2&3 CLASS

Four-Day

Facilitated by Gary Douglas, the founder of Access, and Dain Heer

These classes invite you to go beyond this reality and generate your life as phenomenal. The lies of this reality pertaining to the love/hate program, you as a victim, the perfection of success, so-called "disabilities," insane relationships, and eternal sadness will be cleared from your universe. You will recognize where you have denied joy and happiness from your life and begin to acknowledge yourself as the valuable product. Your talents and abilities will continue to be uncovered, as well as your communion with your body. Choose to step into the potency of allowance and oneness to create change on the planet. Claim the magic that you can create in your life and for others.

Prerequisites: Bars Class, Foundation & One

www.AccessConsciousness.com

ACCESS BODY CLASS

Varies

In this dynamic hands on class you will receive and gift hands on body processes which will shift your body from degenerating itself into generating itself. The processes you learn will create your body and those of your friends and family, to function with more ease and joy. Those attending this class report few sicknesses, less pain, and an easier ability to create the body they desire. What would it take for you and your body to be in communion? What else is possible?

www.AccessConsciousness.com

INFORMATION

For more information on Gary Douglas, Dr. Dain Heer, books and other products; Access Energy Transformation seminars, workshops or classes; class registrations or if you have any questions please visit:

www.AccessConsciousness.com

OTHER ACCESS WEB SITE

www.DrDainHeer.com

www.GaryMDouglas.com

www.Facebook.com/accessconsciousness

www.Twitter.com/accessconscious

www.ConsciousHorseConsciousRider.com

www.RightRecoveryForYou.com

www.AccessTrueKnowledgeFoundation.com

www.MySpace.com/accessconsciousness

www.Costarricense-Paso.com

Printed in Great Britain
by Amazon.co.uk, Ltd.,
Marston Gate.